The Sick Bug
Goes to School

by Susie Bazil

Illustrated by Shawn McCann

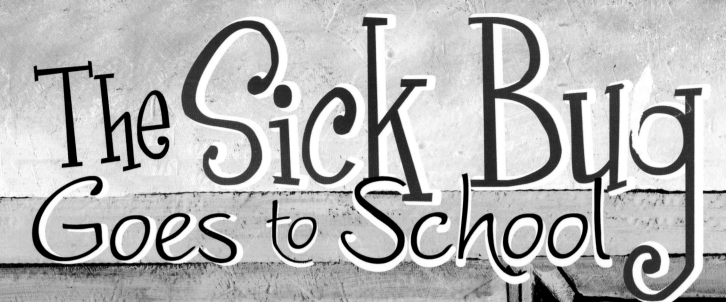
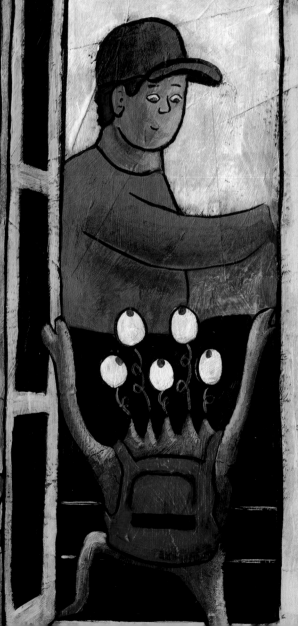
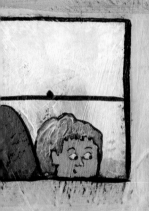
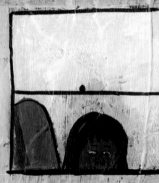
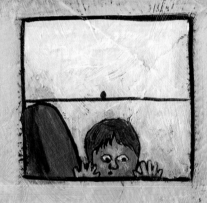
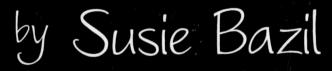
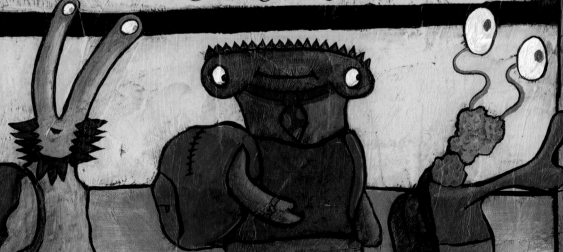

Illustrations by Shawn McCann

www.thesickbug.com

ISBN 10: 1-59298-346-4
ISBN 13: 978-1-59298-346-9

Library of Congress Catalog Number: 2010935823

Printed in the United States of America
First Printing: 2011

15   14   13   12   11   5   4   3   2   1

Cover and interior design by James Monroe Design, LLC.

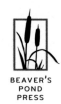

BEAVER'S
POND
PRESS

Beaver's Pond Press, Inc.
7104 Ohms Lane, Suite 101
Edina, MN 55439-2129
(952) 829-8818
www.beaverspondpress.com

To order, visit www.BeaversPondBooks.com or call 1-800-901-3480.
Reseller discounts available.

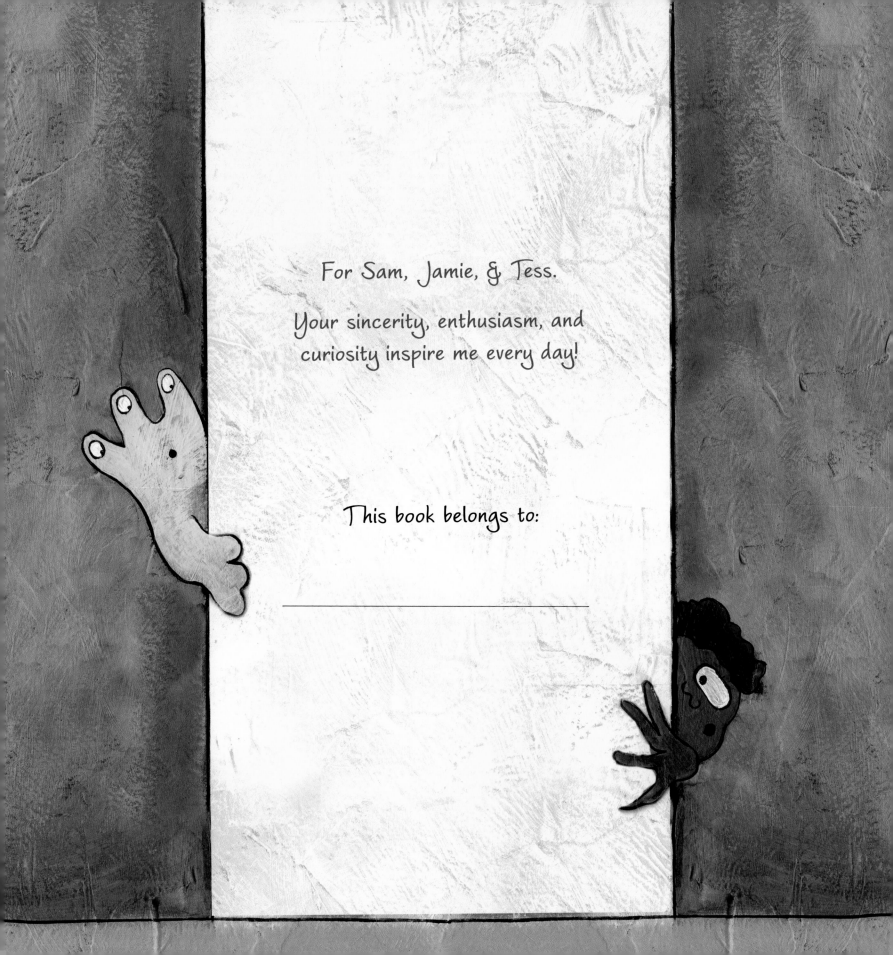

For Sam, Jamie, & Tess.

Your sincerity, enthusiasm, and
curiosity inspire me every day!

This book belongs to:

_____

The school doors flew open one day in the fall,
and busses brought children who ran through the halls.

The kids made new friends and they learned how to spell,
but one day in Room 8, Jamie didn't feel well.

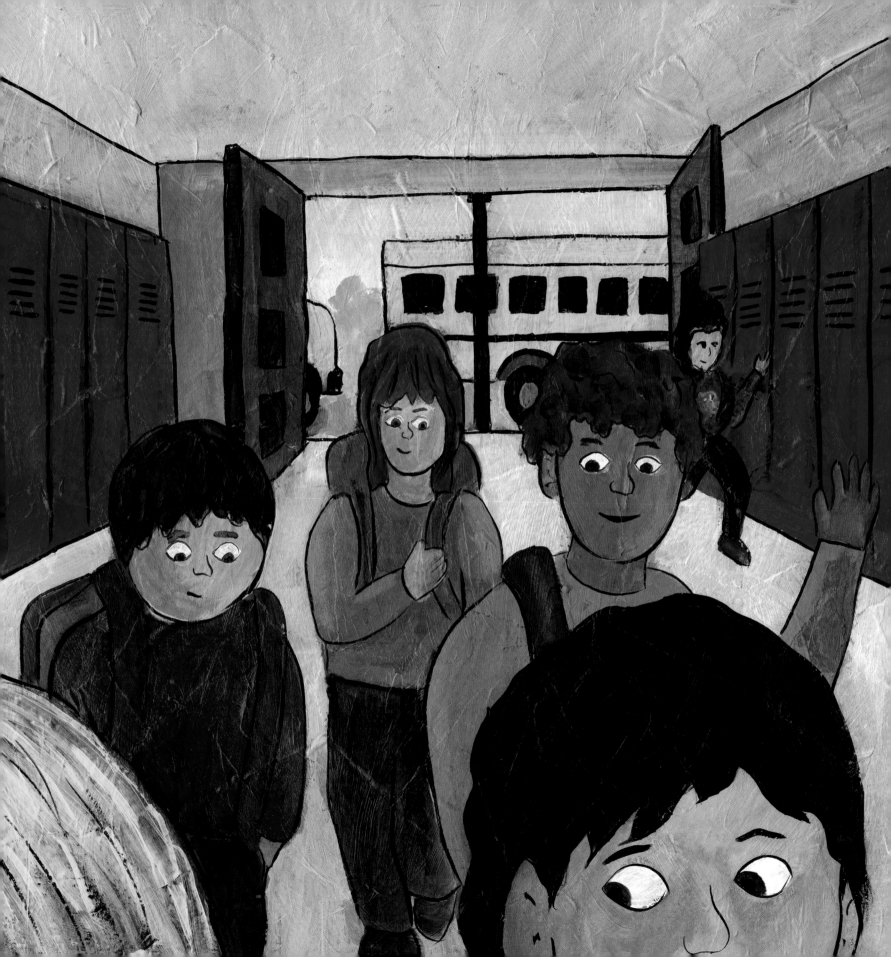

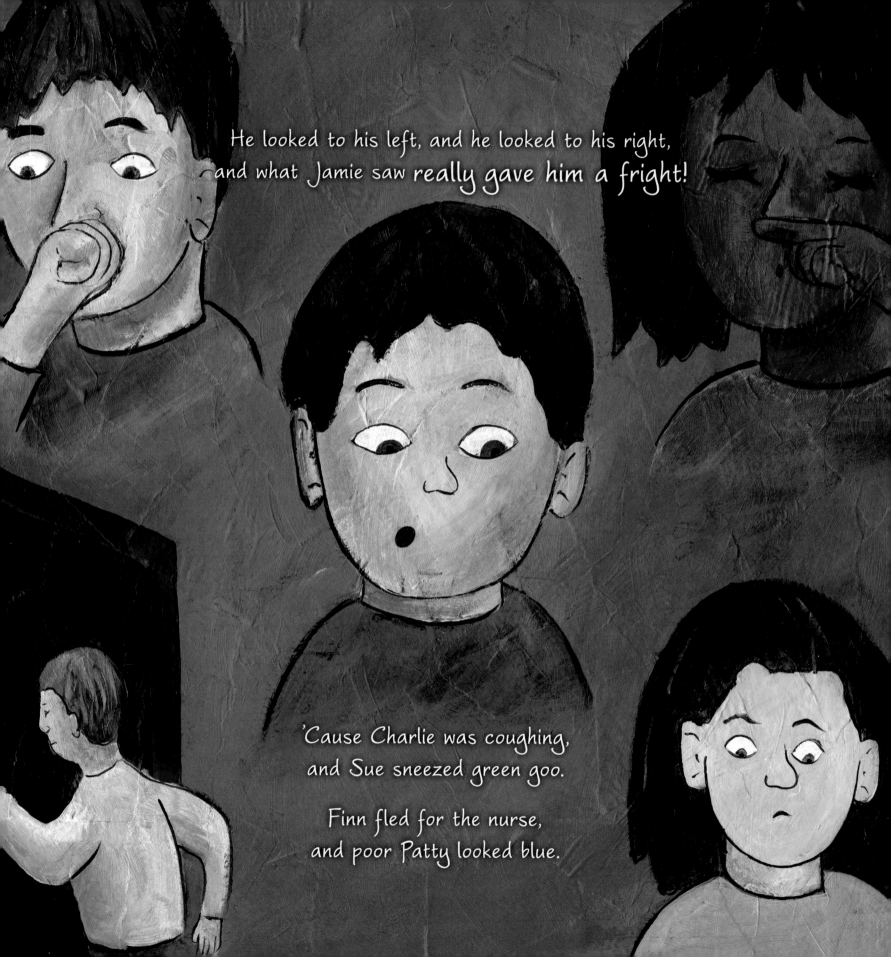

He looked to his left, and he looked to his right,
and what Jamie saw really gave him a fright!

'Cause Charlie was coughing,
and Sue sneezed green goo.

Finn fled for the nurse,
and poor Patty looked blue.

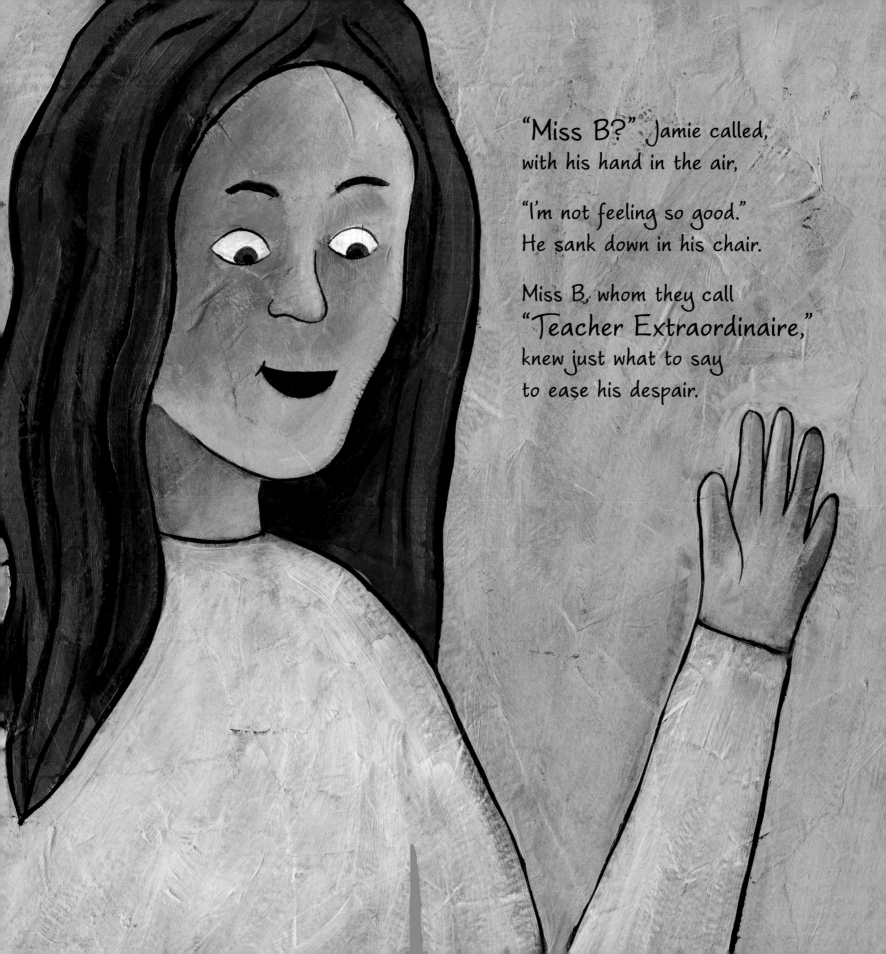

"Miss B?" Jamie called,
with his hand in the air,

"I'm not feeling so good."
He sank down in his chair.

Miss B, whom they call
"Teacher Extraordinaire,"
knew just what to say
to ease his despair.

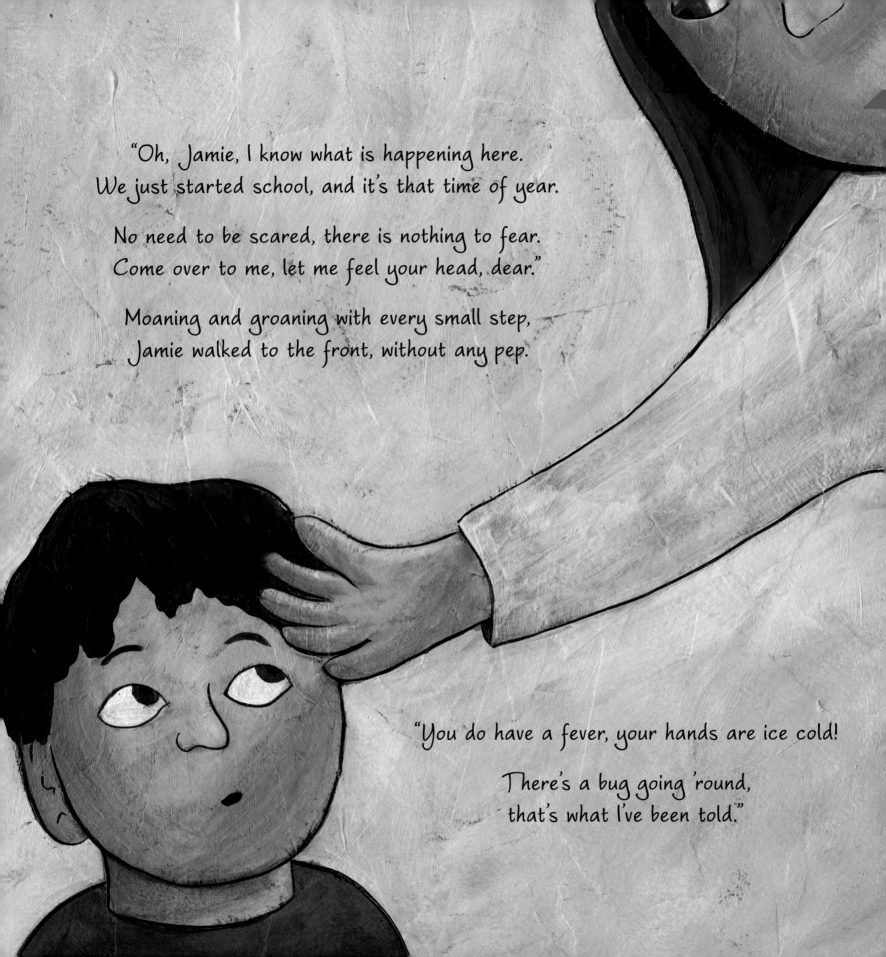

"Oh, Jamie, I know what is happening here.
We just started school, and it's that time of year.

No need to be scared, there is nothing to fear.
Come over to me, let me feel your head, dear."

Moaning and groaning with every small step,
Jamie walked to the front, without any pep.

"You do have a fever, your hands are ice cold!

There's a bug going 'round,
that's what I've been told."

Today's Schedule

Writers Workshop
Reading
MATH
RECESS
LUNCH
Read to Self
Gym
Snack

CLASS RULES

RAISE HANDS FIRST
BE POLITE TO OTHERS
NO BUGS or PETS
Homework before play

"A bug in our class?
There's no bugs in our school!"

Jamie's voice rang out loud as he read the class rules.

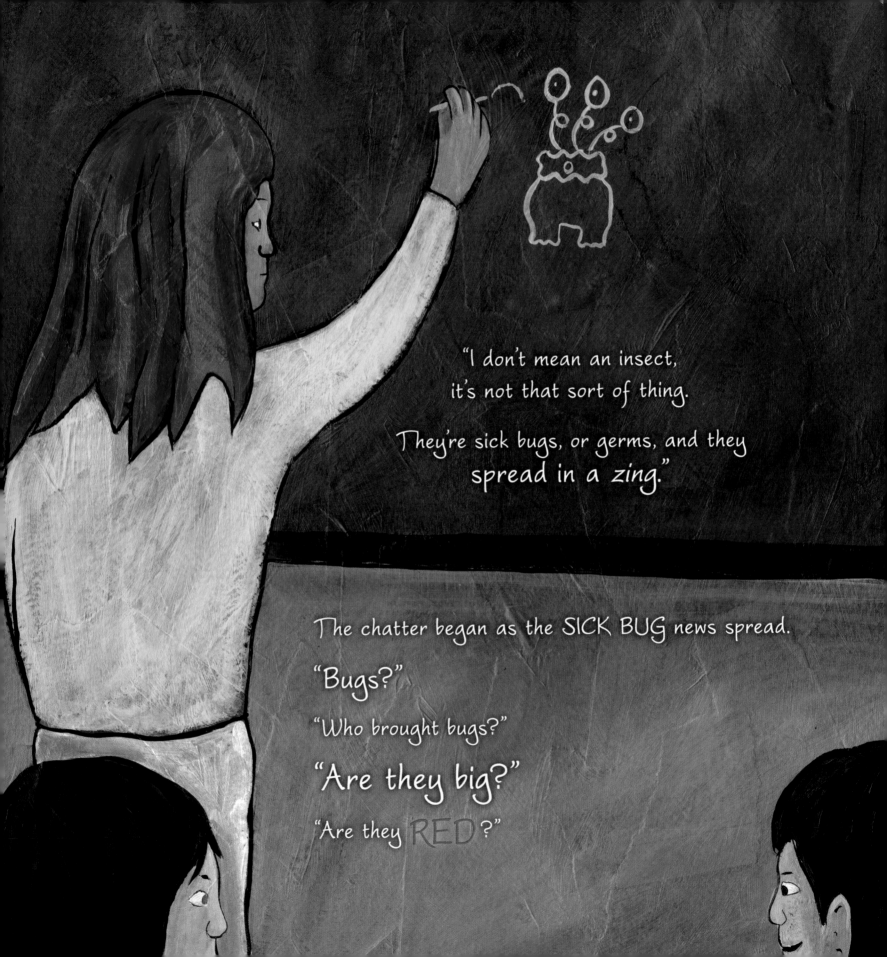

"I don't mean an insect,
it's not that sort of thing.

They're sick bugs, or germs, and they
spread in a zing."

The chatter began as the SICK BUG news spread.

"Bugs?"

"Who brought bugs?"

"Are they big?"

"Are they RED?"

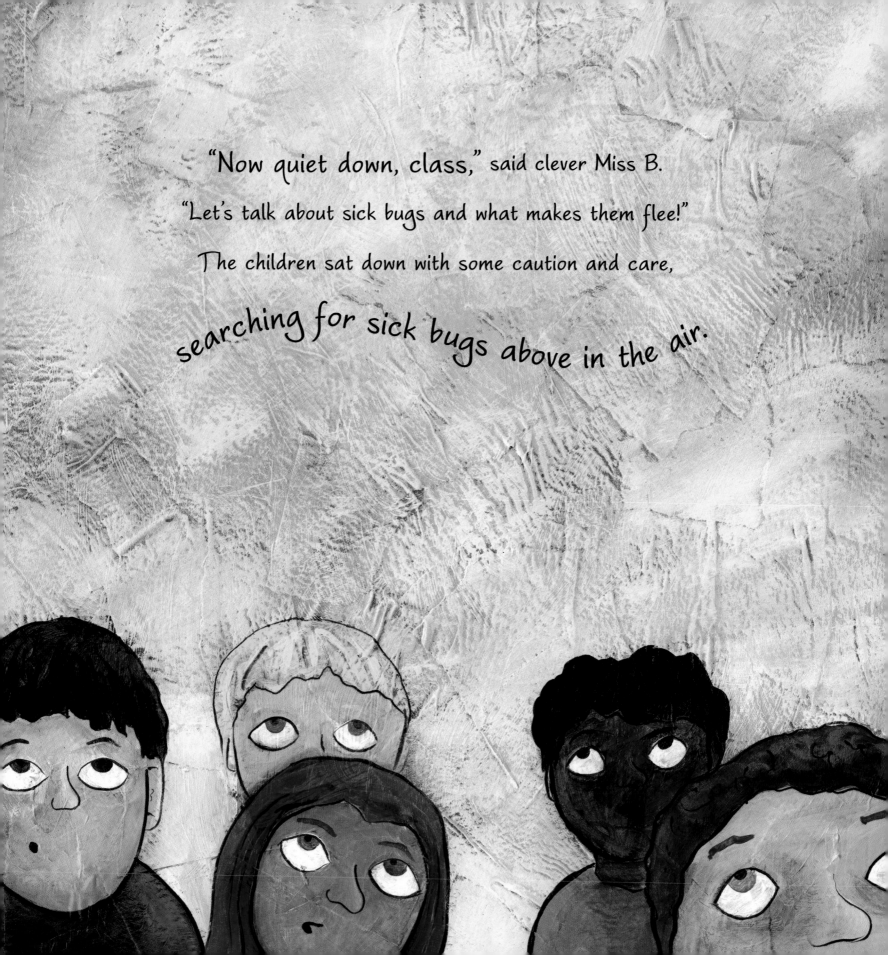

"Now quiet down, class," said clever Miss B.

"Let's talk about sick bugs and what makes them flee!"

The children sat down with some caution and care,

searching for sick bugs above in the air.

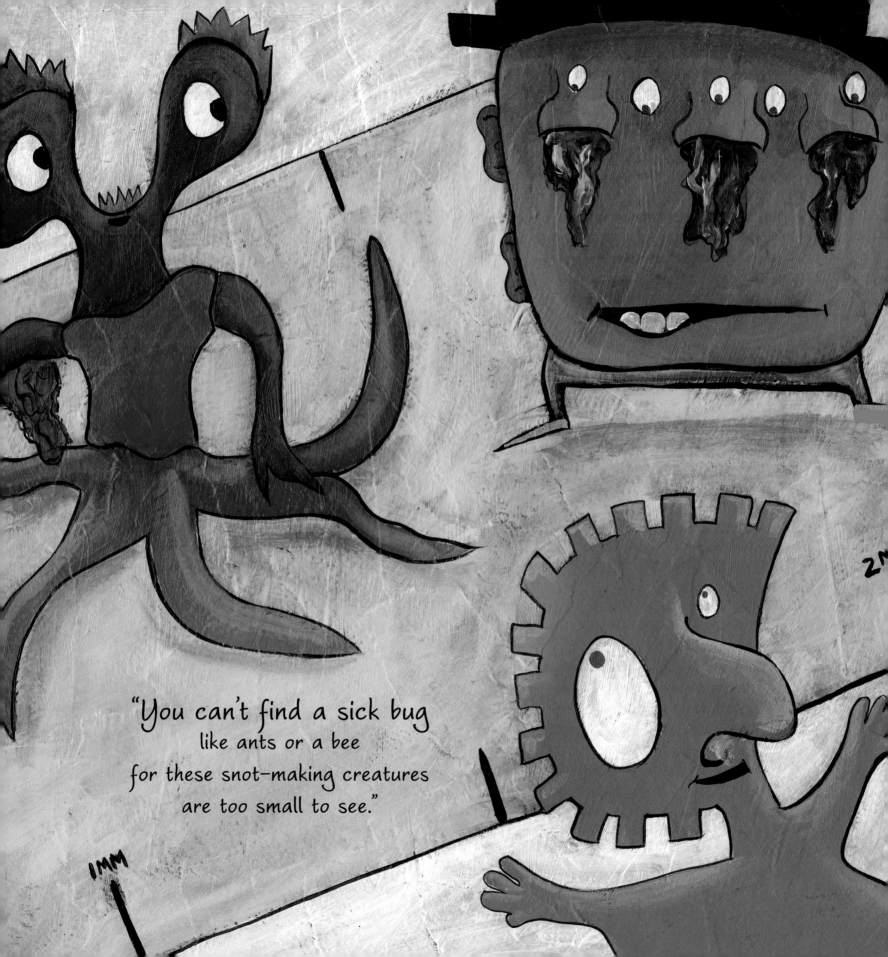

"You can't find a sick bug
like ants or a bee
for these snot-making creatures
are too small to see."

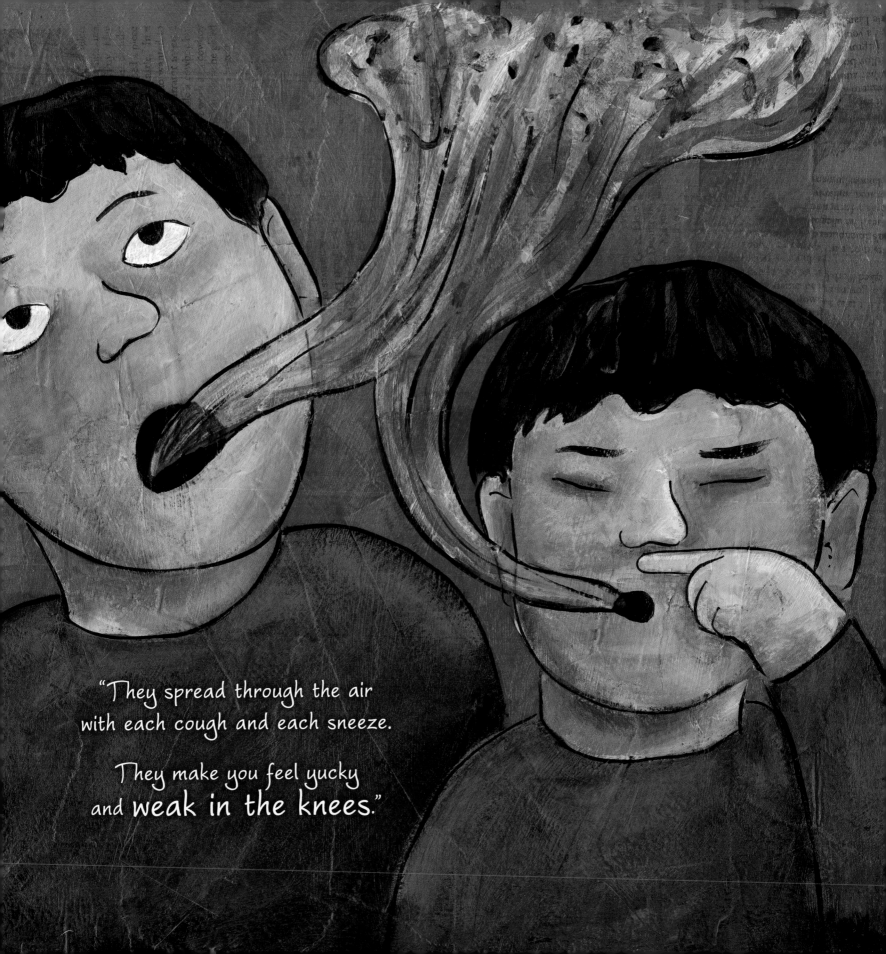

"They spread through the air
with each cough and each sneeze.

They make you feel yucky
and **weak in the knees.**"

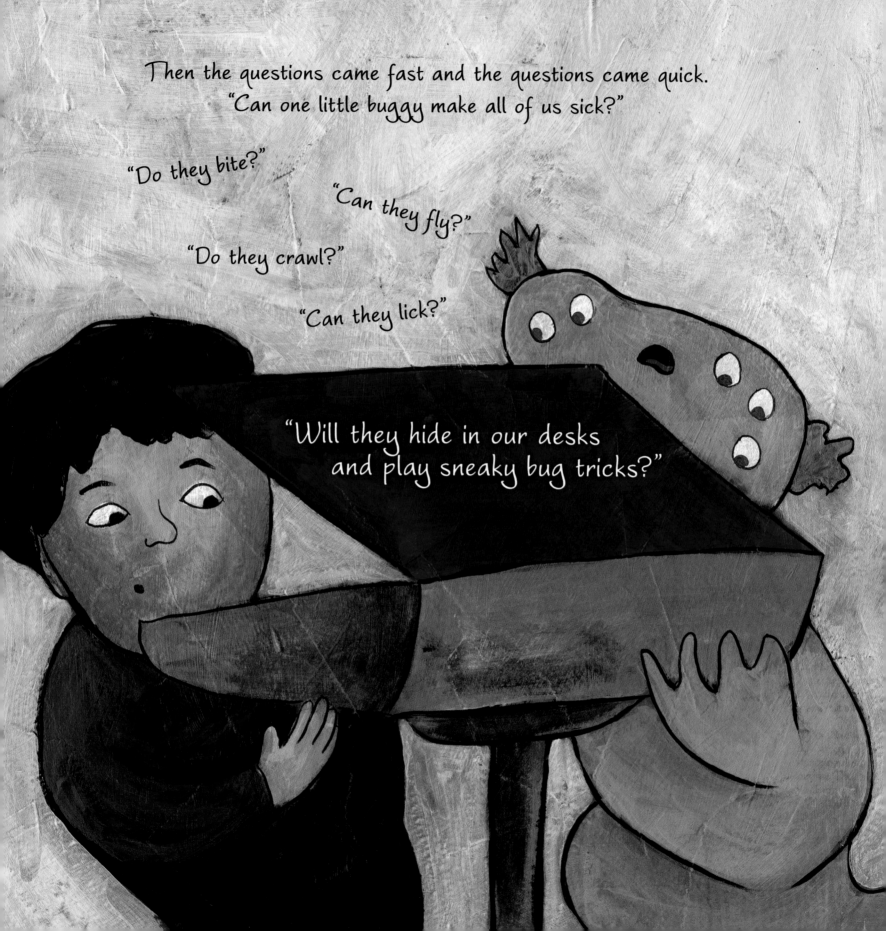

Then the questions came fast and the questions came quick.
"Can one little buggy make all of us sick?"

"Do they bite?"

"Can they fly?"

"Do they crawl?"

"Can they lick?"

"Will they hide in our desks
and play sneaky bug tricks?"

"Let's see," Miss B said with a smile in her eyes.

"You're on the right track—they're like bug super-spies!

I don't think they bite, but they do like to hide.

And if one sick bug finds you, soon more will arrive."

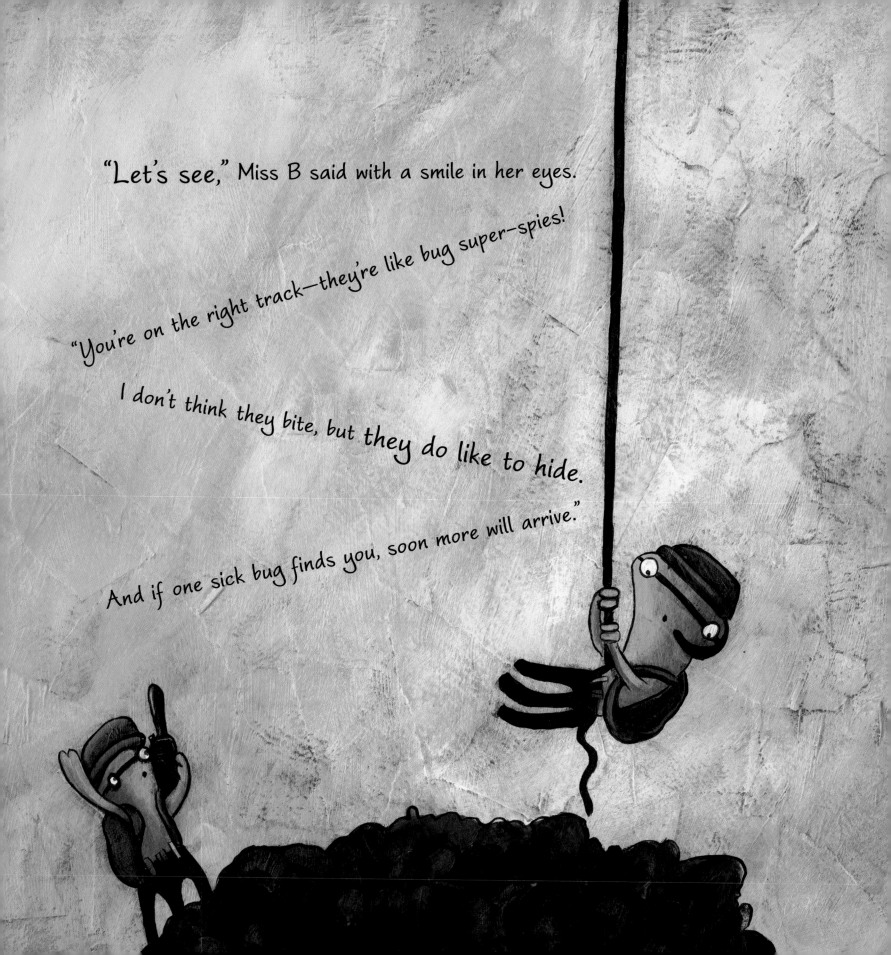

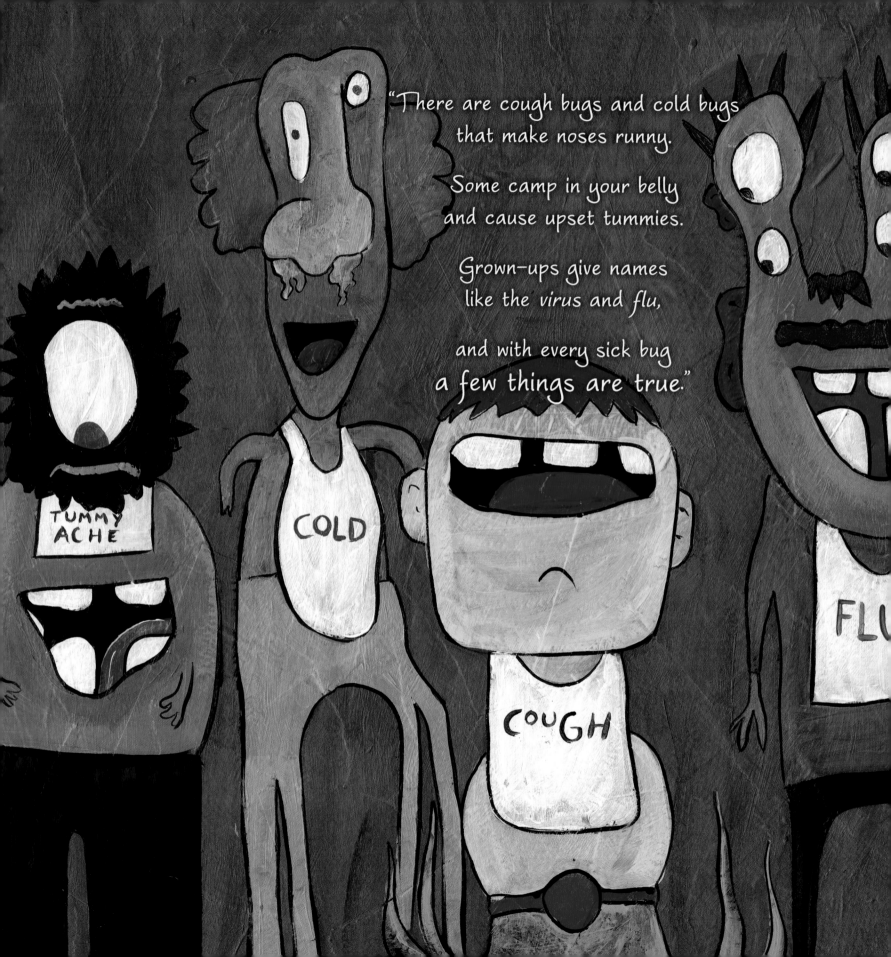

"There are cough bugs and cold bugs
that make noses runny.

Some camp in your belly
and cause upset tummies.

Grown-ups give names
like the virus and flu,

and with every sick bug
a few things are true."

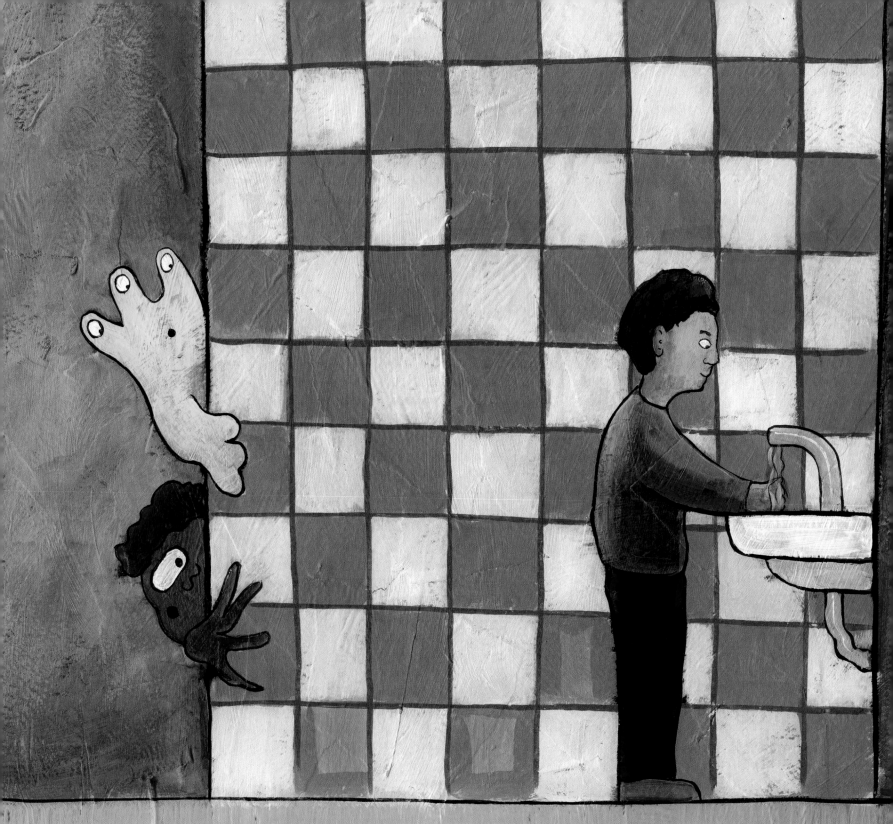

"First, sick bugs are patient and happy to wait
for kids who forget to wash their hands and face."

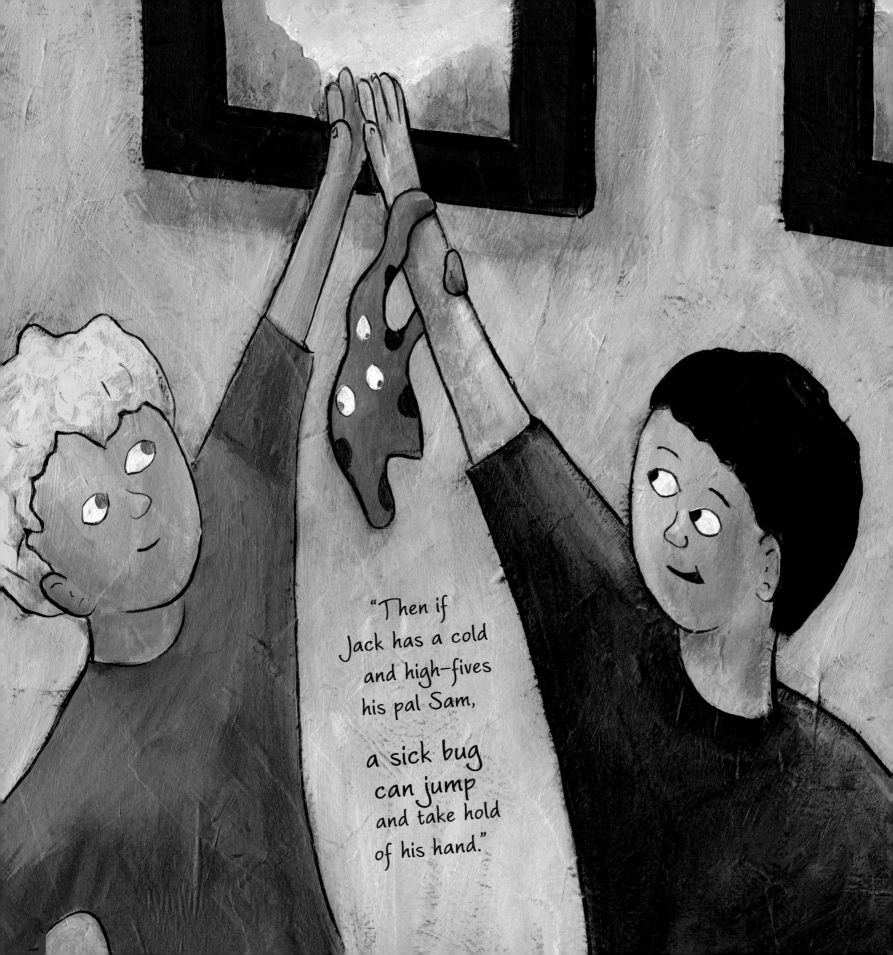

"Then if
Jack has a cold
and high-fives
his pal Sam,

a sick bug
can jump
and take hold
of his hand."

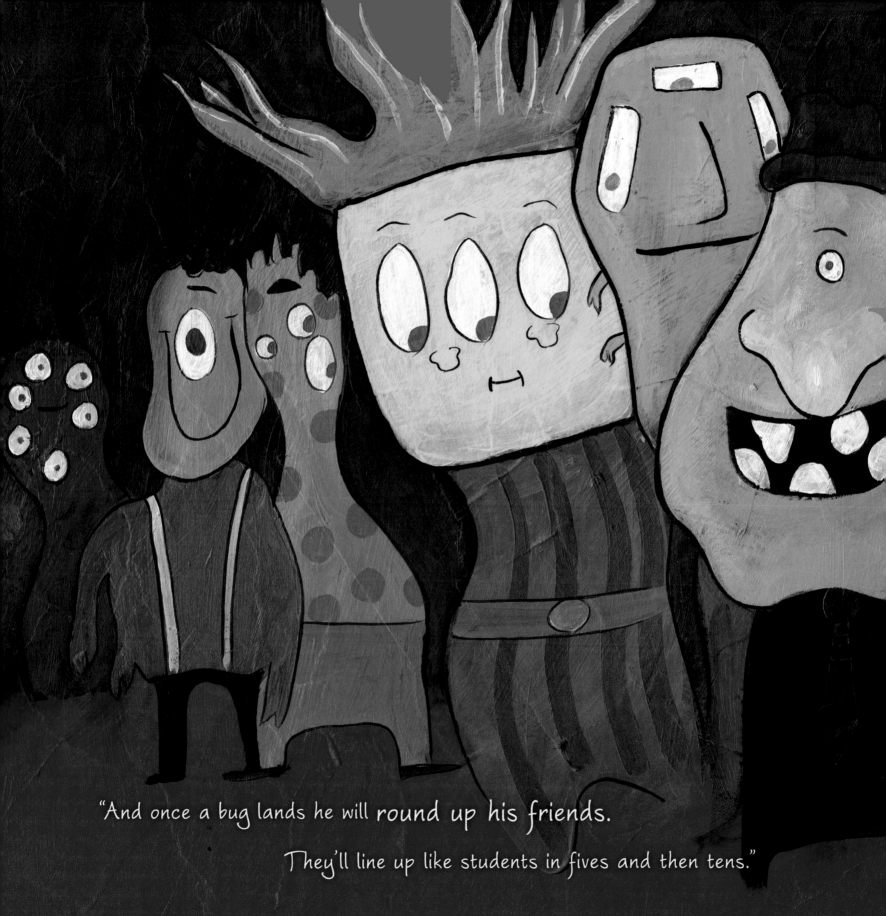

"And once a bug lands he will round up his friends.

They'll line up like students in fives and then tens."

"Then they play leap frog all over the place,

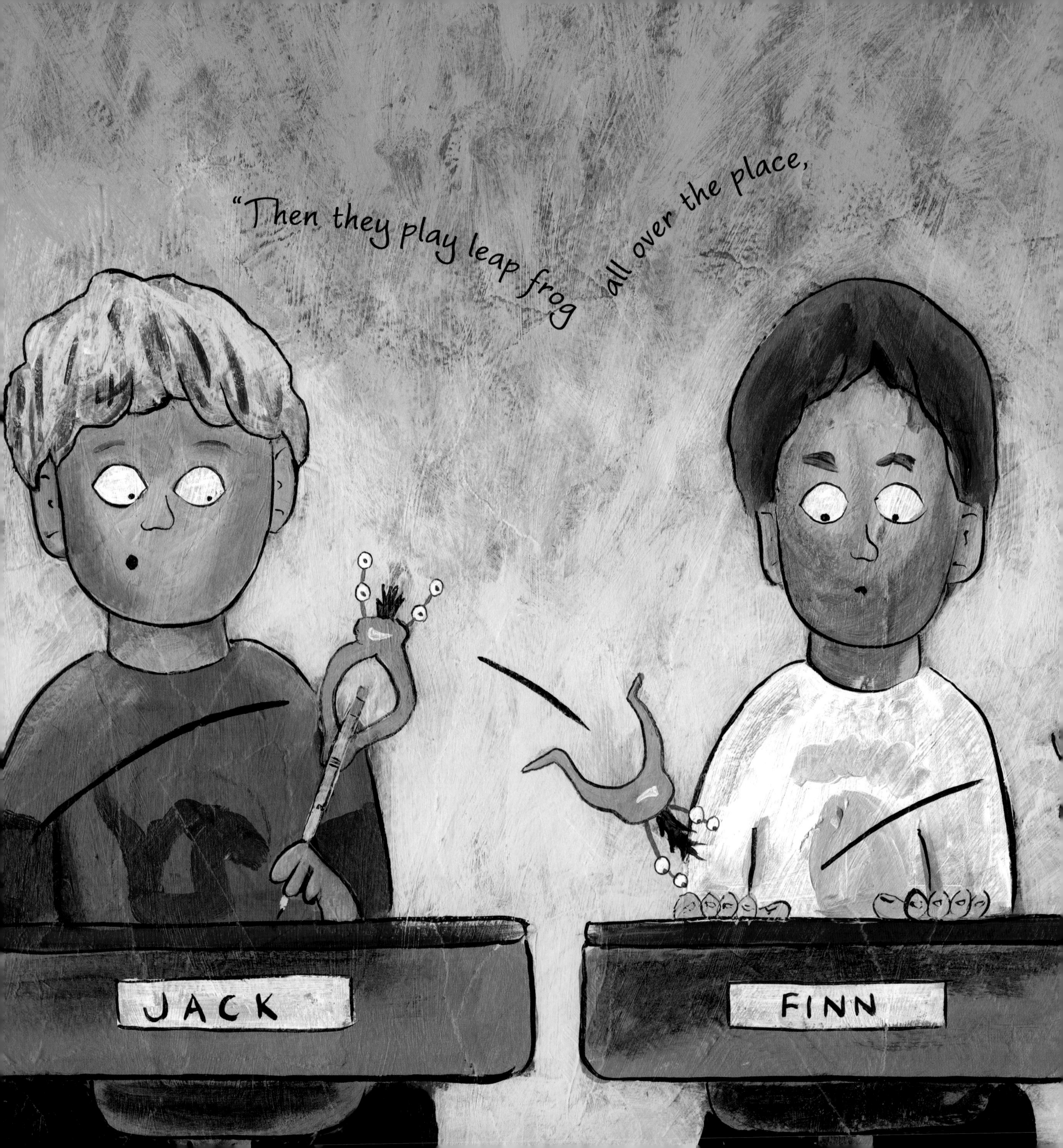

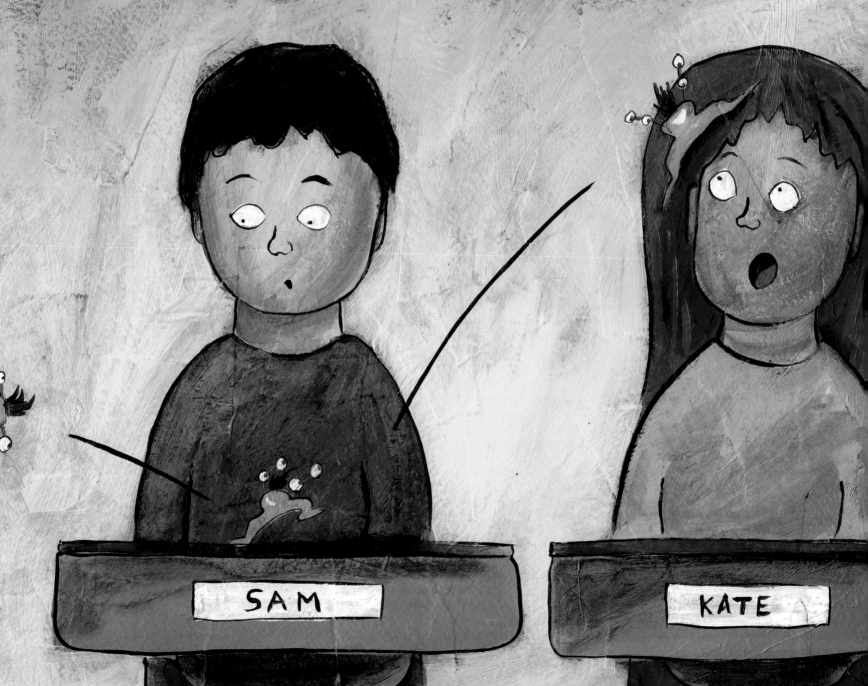

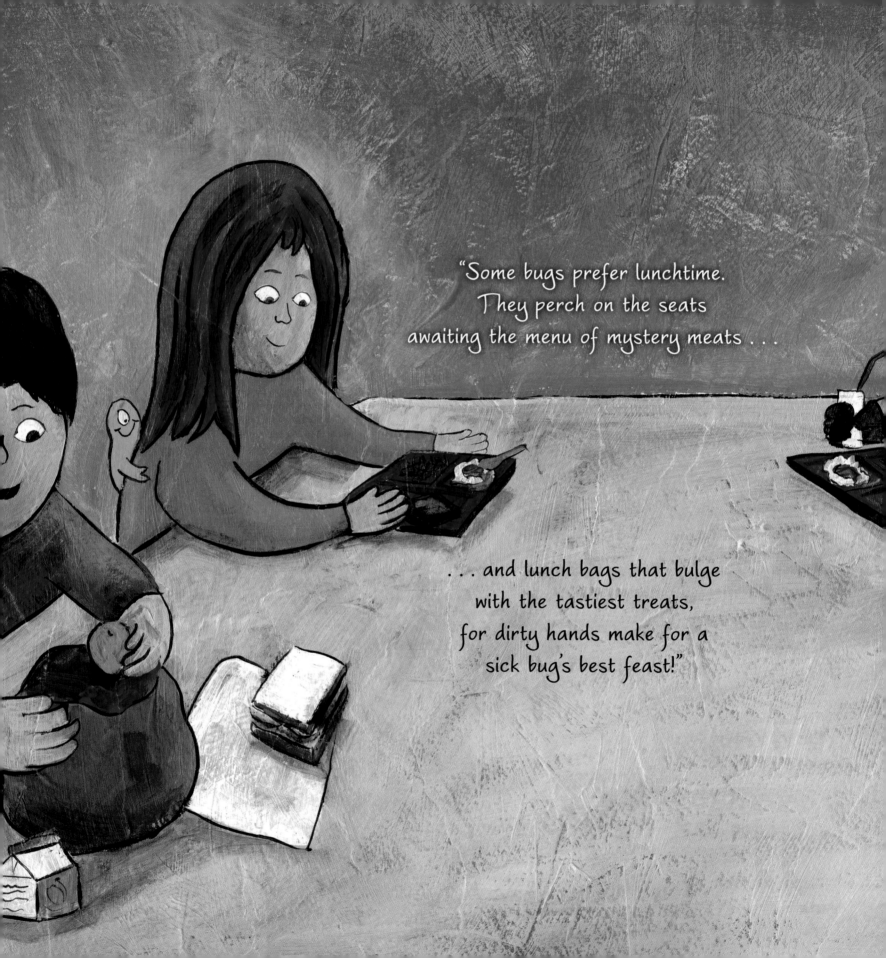

"Some bugs prefer lunchtime.
They perch on the seats
awaiting the menu of mystery meats . . .

. . . and lunch bags that bulge
with the tastiest treats,
for dirty hands make for a
sick bug's best feast!"

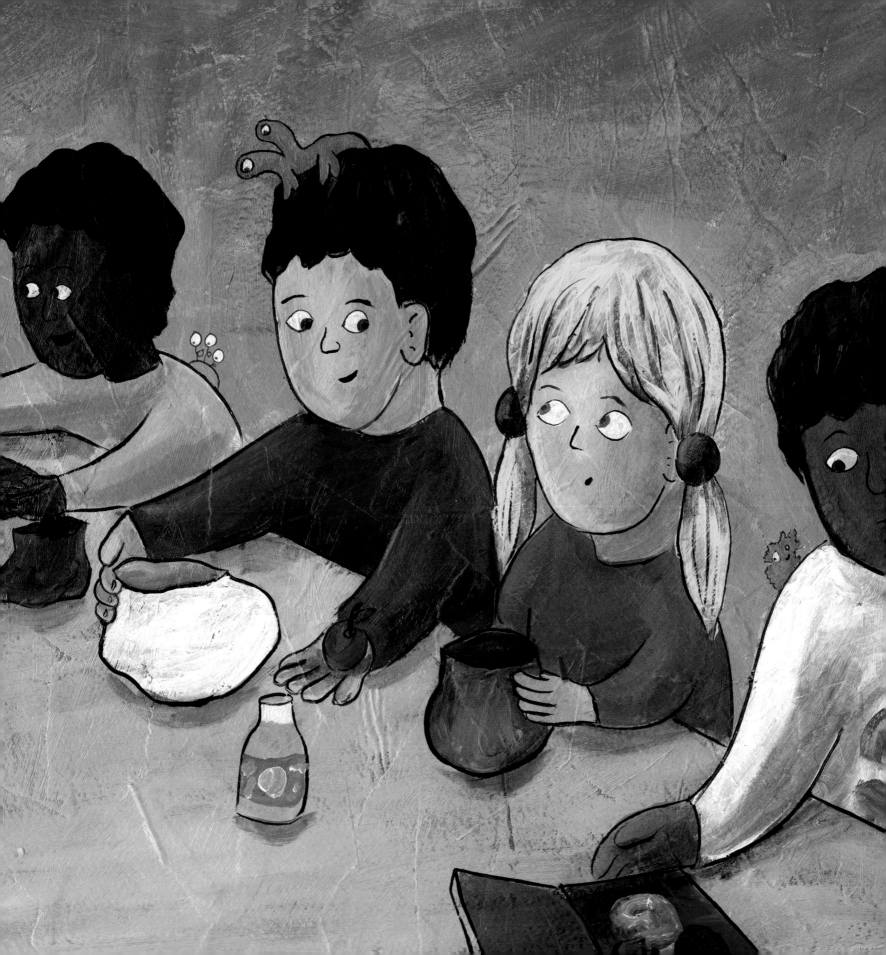

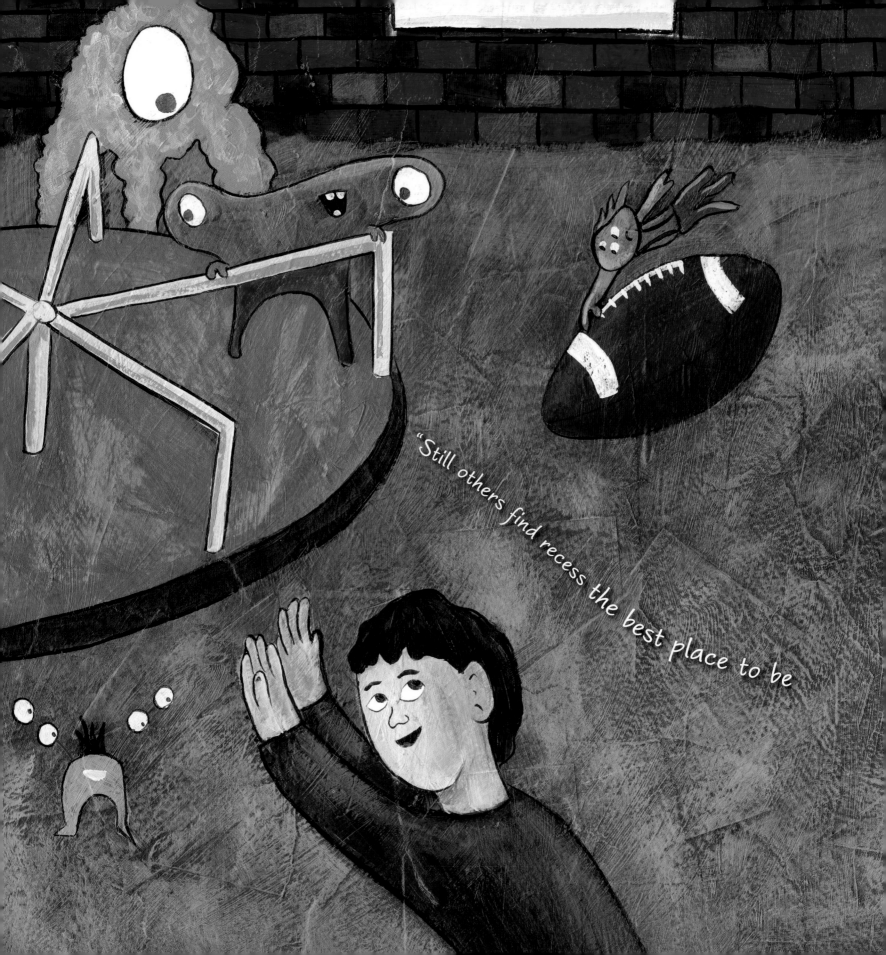

"Still others find recess the best place to be

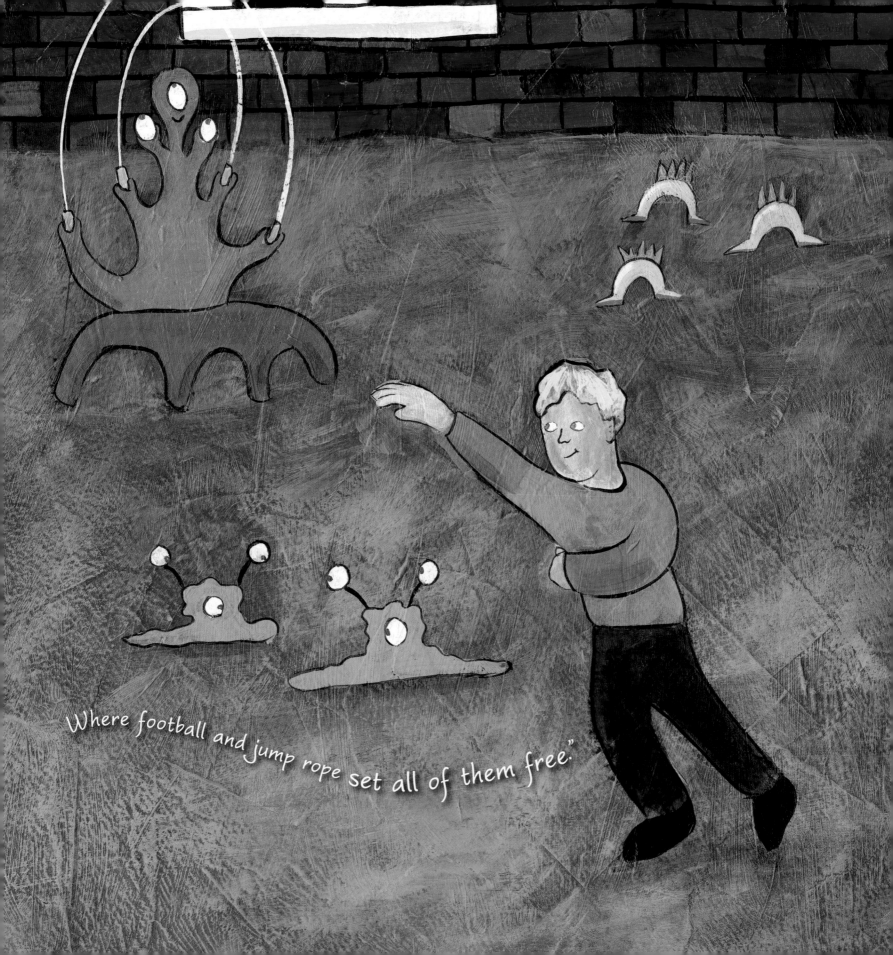

Where football and jump rope set all of them free."

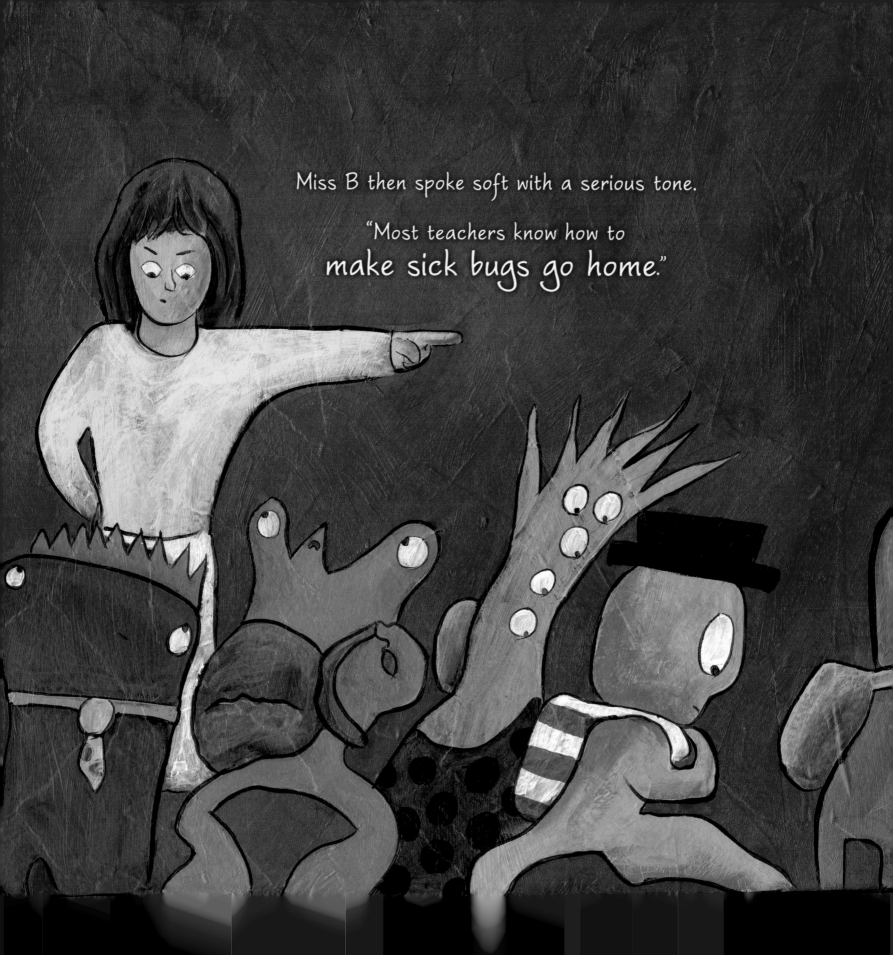

Miss B then spoke soft with a serious tone.

"Most teachers know how to
make sick bugs go home."

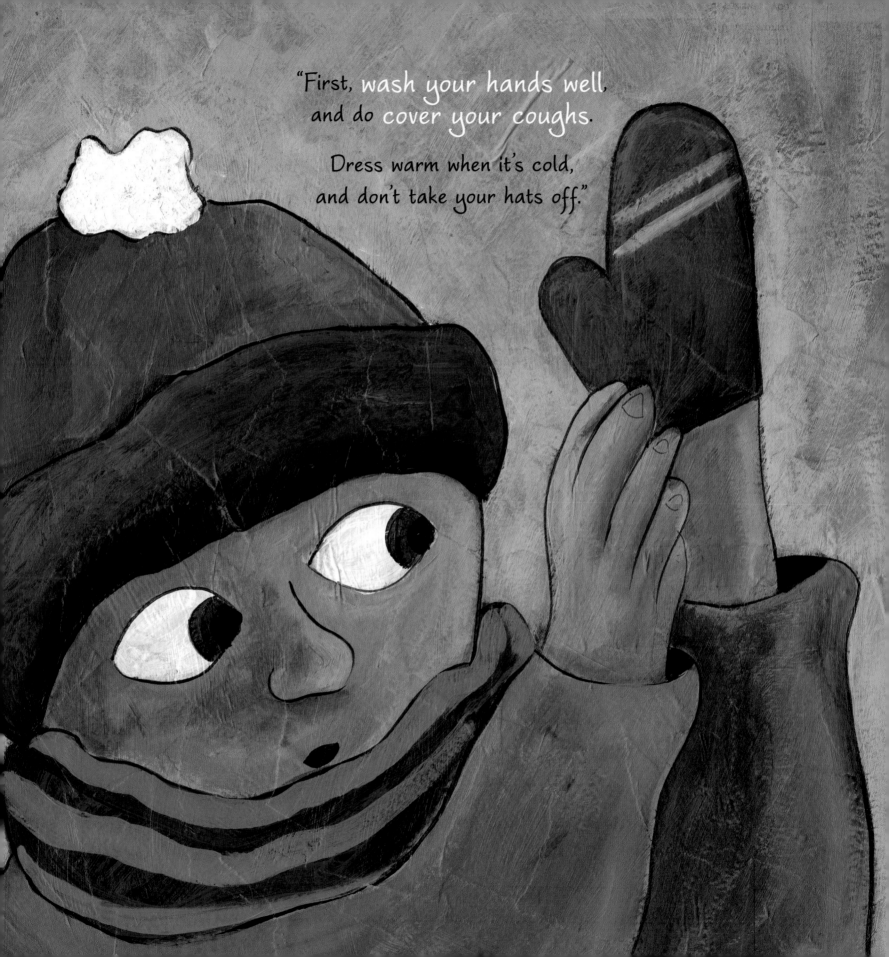

"First, wash your hands well,
and do cover your coughs.

Dress warm when it's cold,
and don't take your hats off."

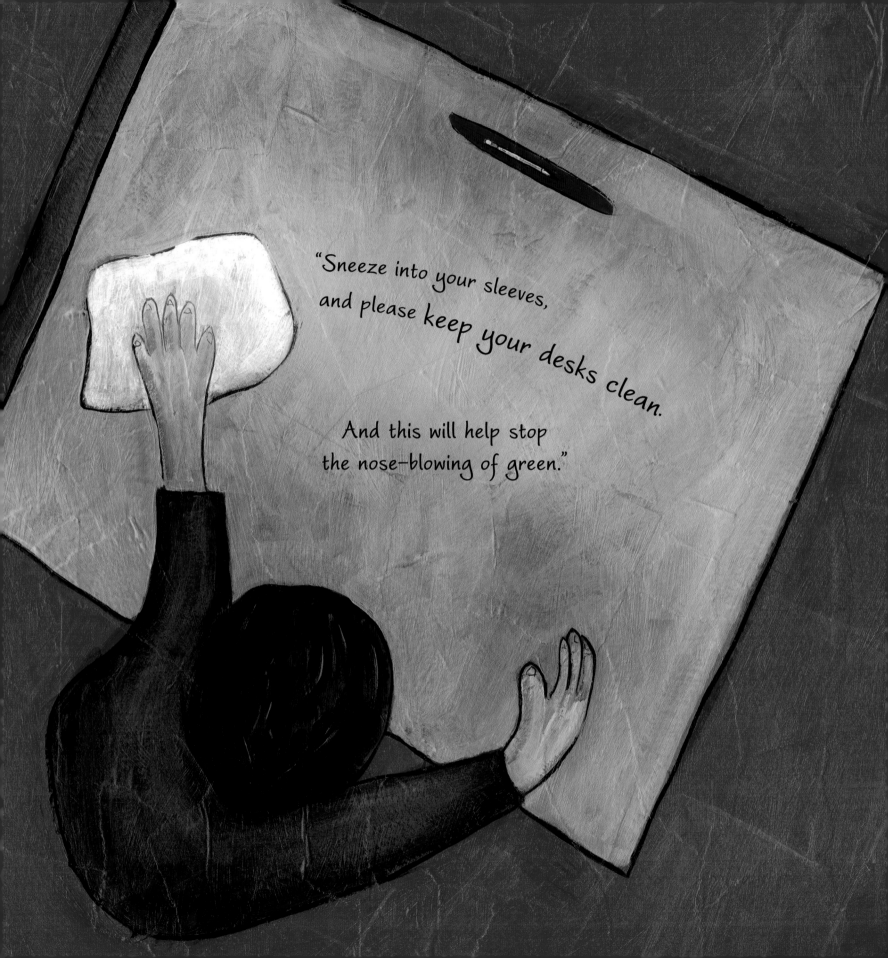

"Sneeze into your sleeves,
and please keep your desks clean.

And this will help stop
the nose-blowing of green."

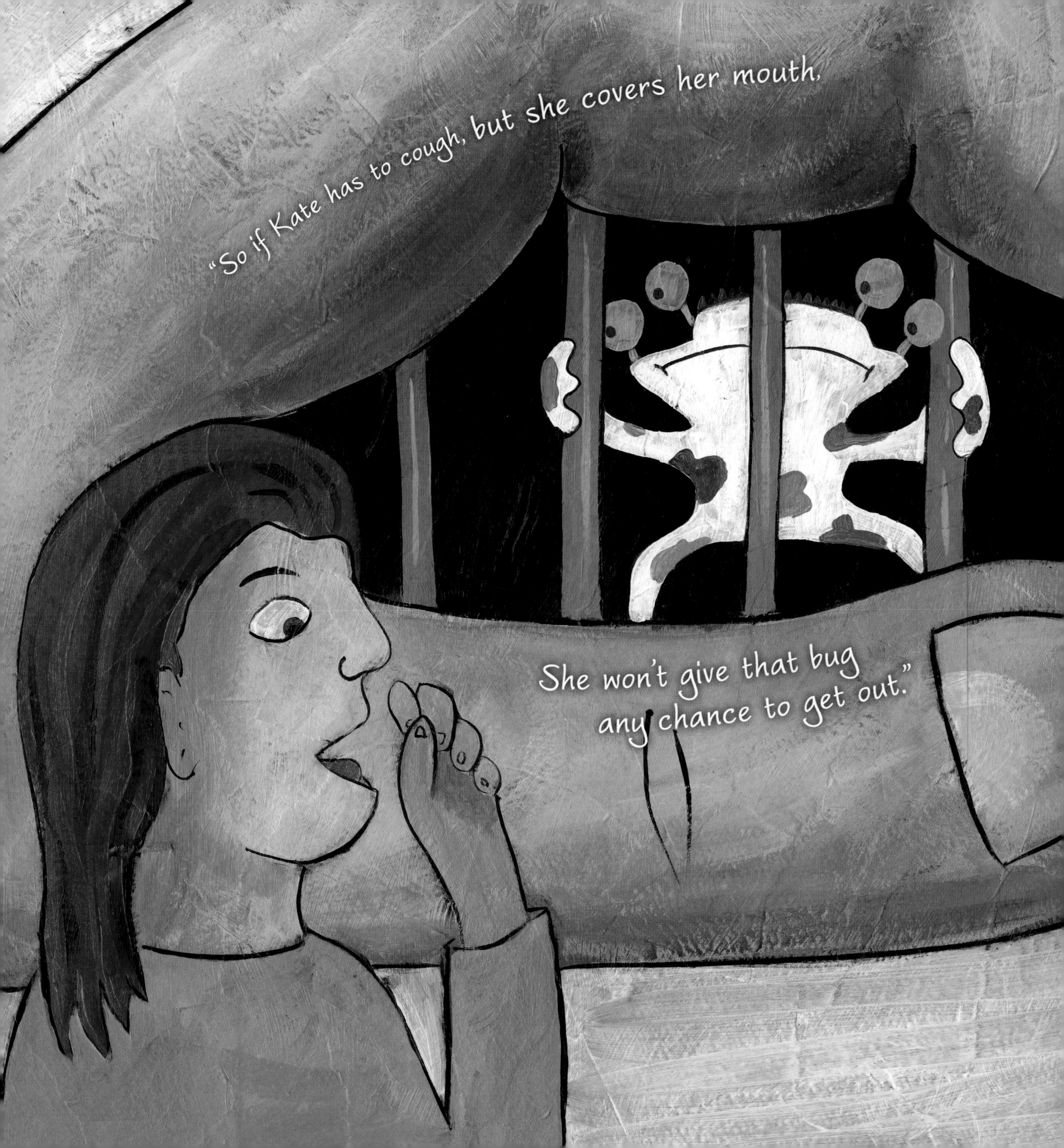

"So if Kate has to cough, but she covers her mouth,

She won't give that bug any chance to get out."

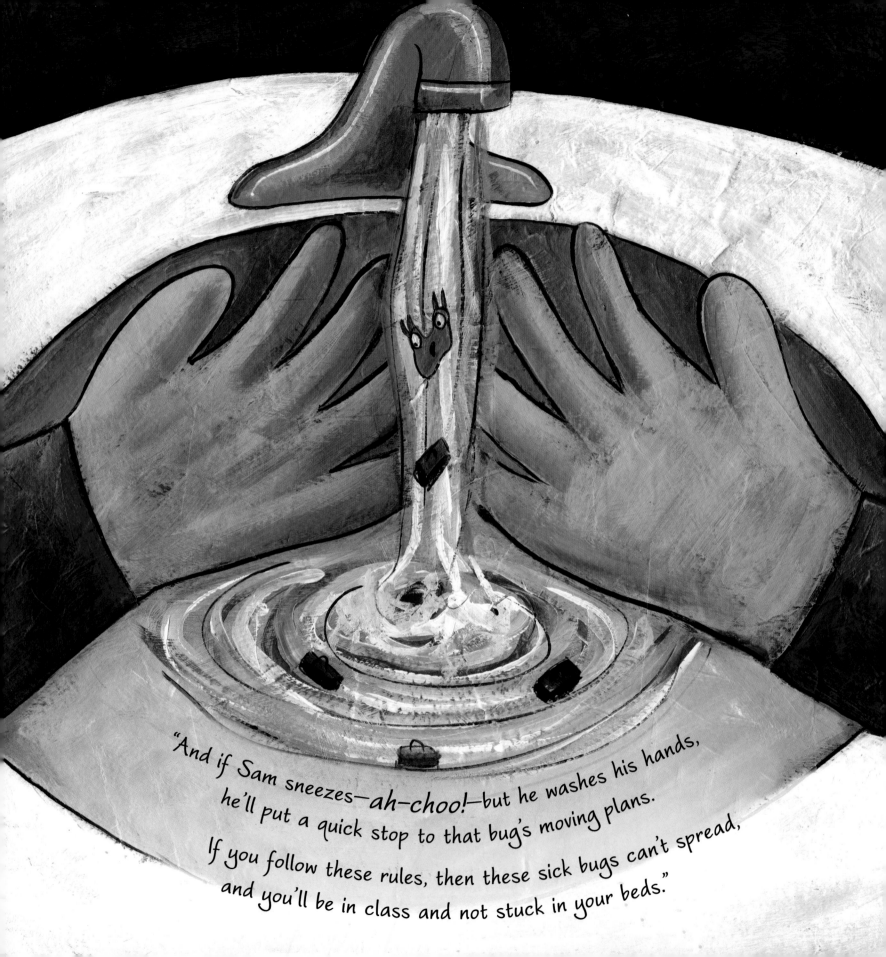

"And if Sam sneezes—*ah-choo!*—but he washes his hands,
he'll put a quick stop to that bug's moving plans.
If you follow these rules, then these sick bugs can't spread,
and you'll be in class and not stuck in your beds."

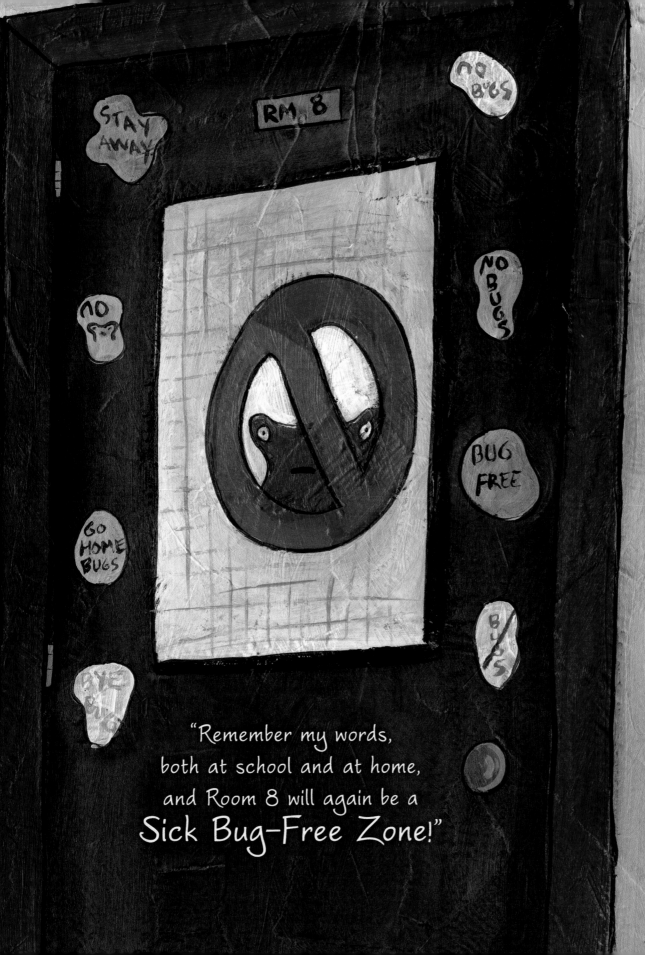

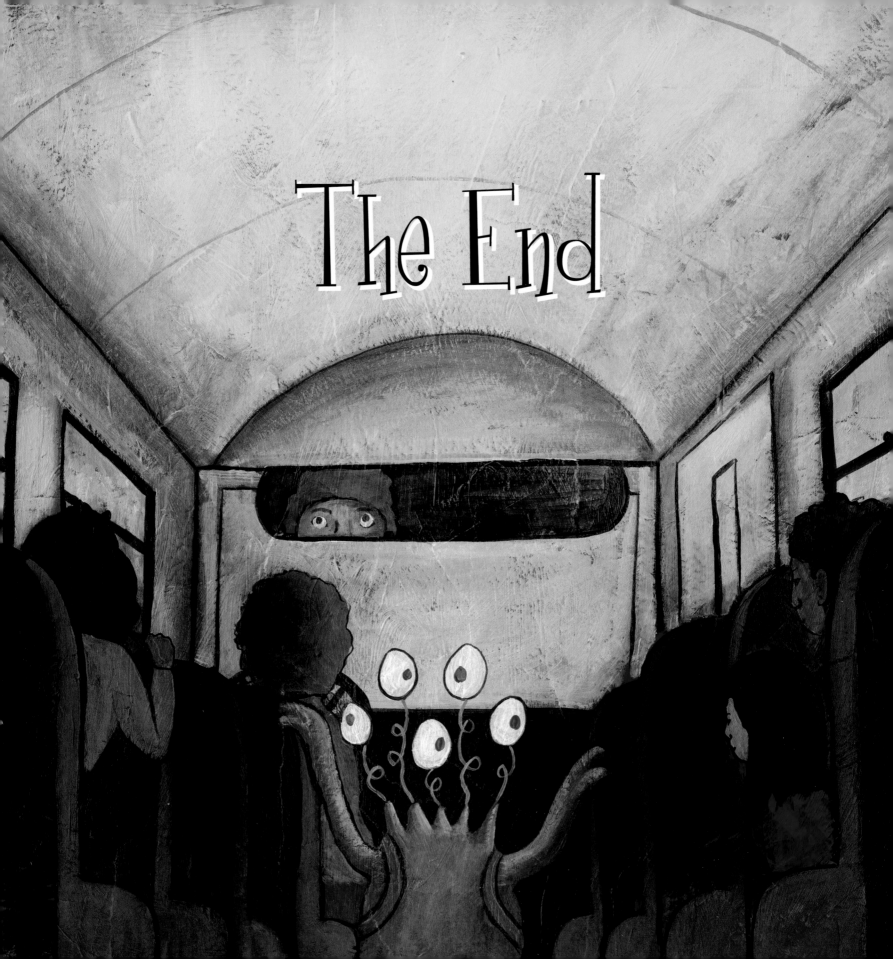